Teaching the Physically Handicapped to Swim

WILLIAM ANDERSON

Diploma, *The Swimming Teachers' Association of Great Britain and the Commonwealth*

Advanced Teachers' Certificate, *The Amateur Swimming Association*

Diploma, *The Royal Life Saving Society*

'Swimming Instructor of the Year' Award for 1951, *The International Federation of Swimming Coaches and Swimming Instructors*

FABER AND FABER
London

First published in 1968
by Faber and Faber Limited
24 Russell Square London WC1
Reprinted 1970
Printed in Great Britain by
Latimer Trend & Co Ltd Plymouth

I.S.B.N. 0 571 08236 X

FOREWORD

Many tributes have been paid to Mr. Anderson through the years and one of the most tangible of these was in 1951, when he was made 'Swimming Instructor of the Year' for his outstanding contribution to convalescent and remedial swimming. This award was given by the International Federation of Swimming Coaches and Swimming Instructors.

Miss Audrey Z. Baker, B.Sc., L.R.C.P., M.R.C.S., Vice-President of the Swimming Teachers' Association, writes:

The author of this small book has made a most valuable contribution to our knowledge of the ways in which water exercises and swimming can be used in the treatment of the disabled. I know of no other book that deals exclusively with this subject or even includes it among other topics.

Mr. Anderson writes from personal experience, in which he has made careful observations over a number of years. The case histories chosen to illustrate his methods are a fascinating revelation of the success that can follow scientific principles intelligently applied to the use of swimming in rehabilitation.

This book should prove indispensable to both physiotherapists and those swimming instructors who undertake this specialized form of teaching. It is greatly hoped that authorities responsible for the building of new swimming baths will bear in mind the recommendations mentioned, because the success of this form of therapy clearly depends both on the skill of the teacher and also in no small measure on the availability of suitable premises and equipment.

Hector Hughes, Esq., Q.C., M.P. for Aberdeen, writes:

It is an honour to commend this work which is idealistic in conception, constructive in method and practical in plan.

I learned to swim as a boy by standing waist-deep in the Irish Sea, striking out till I reached bottom and then beginning all over again. Since then many seas, Scottish, Irish and English, have embraced me as friends and given me health and pleasure. For the disabled that is not so easy. This book is written for them in a skilful way. There are, however, others in need. People in cities, villages and slums far from seas, ponds and rivers who, though able-bodied, cannot swim because they lack opportunity or, perhaps, physical or mental initiative. This book may inspire them. If so, they also may benefit from the author's wide scope and meticulous care.

If he teaches them to swim
Yield gratitude to him
In sea or pond or brook
For his helpful little book.

For all these reasons I congratulate the author and commend his book.

Alfred A. Laverick, Esq., M.I.B.M., A.I.M.Ent., Manager of the Baths for the Warrington County Borough, writes:

It has been said that 'learning to swim is the most rewarding achievement in a person's life', but just what it means to a physically disabled person is hard to imagine. I have been associated, in an administrative capacity, with the author, in the work he describes, for eighteen years and have watched with interest, and often with amazement, the progress of his pupils.

The author, in writing of his knowledge and experience in this specialized field of swimming tuition, is rendering a valuable service to those who are physically disabled.

CONTENTS

ILLUSTRATIONS

Plates

Figures

PREFACE

Swimming is acknowledged to be the finest form of physical education, and the best means towards physical rehabilitation.

Human affliction is universal, and although the purpose of this book is primarily for the guidance of teachers of swimming, physiotherapists, physical educationists and those who are concerned with the disabled, I hope that it will appeal to all who have regular contact with swimming. Attention to this branch of instruction is, in a general sense, neglected. More prominence and wider publicity could be given to it by national bodies that govern swimming in various countries, encouraging clubs and kindred organizations to promote and establish classes where it can be practised and its effective value recognized.

Education Authorities and voluntary societies for the physically handicapped would be able to organize weekly sessions where those in their care could experience the joy of shedding for a while the encumbrance of braces and calipers, with the ultimate prospect of learning to swim. I have been prompted to compile this manual in response to many inquiries, some from overseas, and through such contact I am able to record that a class for the physically handicapped was successfully established in Canada.

Often I am asked, 'What approach would you use to teach a physically disabled person to swim?' The disabilities that are listed have been encountered by me during twenty years' experience in teaching the physically disabled (mostly children) to swim, and the methods of instruction described are those which I have used and proved to be effective. I do not claim that they are the best, as I have never seen any others demonstrated or described. What I do claim however is that they have produced remarkable and gratifying results, and trust that they will be of some guidance to those who are beset with similar problems. Should my work simply evoke criticism and discussion it will have served a useful purpose, for out of a controversy over a subject like this, only goodness and improvement can emerge.

W. A.

ACKNOWLEDGEMENTS

I wish to record my grateful thanks to Audrey Z. Baker, B.Sc., L.R.C.P., M.R.C.S., for her helpful guidance and advice in the preparation of this book, for the very generous assistance that I have been privileged to receive from her in the past, and for the inspiration I have found through her kind encouragement.

It is a natural consequence for Hector Hughes, Esq., Q.C., M.P., to interest himself in my book. As well as being a regular daily swimmer for many years, he is also a great campaigner on behalf of the swimming fraternity and the need for improved facilities, especially the provision of more swimming pools. With great appreciation I record to him my sincere thanks for granting to me the privilege and generosity of his kind support.

Mr. A. A. Laverick, M.I.B.M., A.I.M.Ent., became acquainted with almost all my pupils. He has watched them undergoing instruction and has seen their progress and ultimate recovery. To him I tender my sincere thanks for the facilities he placed at our disposal, and for his many expressions of encouragement to my pupils and myself.

I would also like to thank Dr. W. H. S. Wallace who helped to edit the manuscript, and Miss Mary Waldron for her line drawings. The photograph of a child learning to swim is published by courtesy of the Manchester *Daily Mail.*

Chapter I

FIRST PRINCIPLES

The treatment of the physically handicapped aims at training them to overcome their disabilities. Although these disabilities may be incurable, training can achieve much to re-establish powers that have been lost. The work of training the physically handicapped to overcome their disabilities is carried out by physiotherapists who have special knowledge of the use of exercises and movements in the development and control of muscular movements. There are two main objectives in the training: one is the development of muscles that have become weak as the result of disuse and the second is to train and develop other muscles that may be used to take over the function of muscles whose use has been lost by injury or disease.

The work of the physiotherapist is supplemented by that of the swimming teacher with his knowledge of swimming strokes and how some movements propel the swimmer, others retard movement and of how balance is learnt. He has the advantage of being able to use water as a medium in which to work as it can be of great assistance in carrying out rehabilitation activities. In water the limbs are supported by its buoyancy and this greatly assists a disabled person to develop his powers to regain control of normal movements. In addition, more muscles are used when swimming than is possible in static exercises and consequently the exercises have greater value. With the rhythm of the swimming stroke, regular breathing is assured, thus developing and strengthening the organs of respiration, which help in promoting a good circulation and strong constitution, while the tonic effect of the water upon the skin produces a feeling of healthy vitality. When teaching a physically handicapped pupil to swim, it is better not to be dogmatic in trying to teach a good style, but rather to remember that regular respiration without any discomfort is what is important and desirable. Never at any time, either during strokes or exercises, should the affected limb be worked beyond its range of power. Style is dependent on power, and power is regulated by the extent of damage sustained by the nerve and muscle fibres.

Style, therefore, is not all-important, and occasionally it is necessary to resort to 'tricks' in order to obtain balance and propulsion. In the breast stroke, for instance, a pupil with a weakened forearm would be encouraged to press and pull with the elbow, and this would affect the style of his legs.

Subsequently style will improve correspondingly as power increases.

When a normal body is at rest in the water, it assumes, due to the buoyancy of the water, a symmetrical position and, with children with paralysis, this symmetry of the body must not be disturbed by teaching an anti-symmetrical stroke such as the side stroke. In this the symmetry of the body is lost and during its action the limbs act unequally both in direction and power. The side stroke, therefore, *must not* be taught to a person suffering from infantile paralysis.

SOME GENERAL ADVICE

1. Do not overwork a pupil, as he soon tires, particularly in the early stages. Vary the activities, allow and encourage plenty of free play.

2. Be ready to applaud his efforts and particularly the acquisition of any new skills which he performs.

3. Be very patient, for some persons respond more quickly than others, depending on the type of affliction and the area affected.

4. Do not expect quick results, learn to persevere with faith and confidence and the rewards of patience and endeavour will come in due time.

5. Swimming lessons should always be augmented by exercises directed towards a particular limb or part of the body, typical examples of which are quoted in the following pages. During the execution of these exercises it will be noted that the buoyancy of the water acts both as an assistant and resistant quantity, relative to the type of exercise performed. There are, of course, many variations, and the swimming teacher will find it profitable to refer to *Pool Exercises* by Bolton and Goodwin, published by E. & S. Livingstone.

If at any time the teacher is doubtful whether a certain stroke or exercise would be beneficial or harmful, he should not experiment, but seek the advice of the doctor or physiotherapist, which I am sure will be readily and freely given. This restores confidence in the teacher, who is, after all, responsible for the care and well-being of his pupil.

Chapter II

DISABILITIES DUE TO PARALYSIS

Fortunately as a result of the almost complete disappearance of poliomyelitis, due to immunization against it, there are now few cases of paralysis among children. The two main types of paralysis that still remain are the cerebral palsies and the muscular dystrophies. Children with cerebral palsy or 'spastic' children are those who have suffered brain injury at birth and those with muscular dystrophy suffer from an inherent defect of development leading to weakness and paralysis of various groups of muscles.

Physically handicapped people naturally feel timid and apprehensive, having no sense of balance. It is very necessary that the teacher should be in very close attendance in the water, giving every assistance and encouragement until such time as the patient is able to manage alone. The teacher must decide whether the lesson is to be one aiming at relaxation or mobilizing or strengthening and he will proceed accordingly. Relaxation should be the theme of the first few lessons, so that teacher and patient can get acquainted, enabling the teacher to observe characteristics of movement, ranging from the easy movement to the difficult and to assess the possibilities of various exercises, whilst the patient also benefits by increasing his confidence. The first entry into the water with the teacher is with a rubber ring support under the armpits and the patient is towed on his back (*see* Fig. 1), encouraged to breathe through his mouth, eyes open, and the teacher keeps up a conversation, preferably on topical subjects unconnected with swimming, thus helping the patient to relax and for a while to forget his affliction.

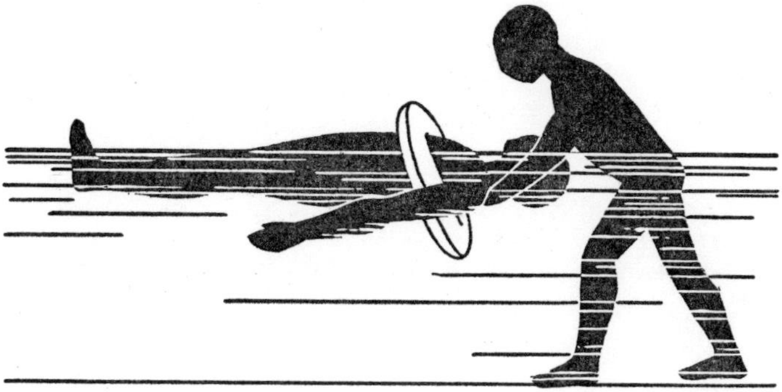

1. On first entering the water, a patient with paralysis is towed on his back by the instructor; a rubber ring is worn under the arm-pits

Where muscles are weakened from any cause it will be noted that other muscles which are associated with the affected ones are not in themselves damaged, but will be found to have lost a certain amount of tone through disuse. Therefore as well as paying attention to the affected ones, the primary exercises should be directed to the restoration of the muscle tone in the unaffected area to normal strength and function. These muscles are then better equipped to support and assist the affected part in its recovery.

Spastic patients are taught in a similar manner to other paralytic patients, but their concentration and co-ordination are usually retarded according to the extent of the affliction. Some are very tensed and are liable to cling tightly to the teacher, others are very nervy and inclined to resist instruction. These moods will, with a little sympathetic understanding and affection, be overcome and the patient will settle down, though progress is usually very slow.

The methods of dealing with different cases of weakness or paralysis may be considered under the headings of the parts of the body affected. It is rare for individual muscles to be paralysed but one part of the body or group of muscles may be affected more than another.

Weakness of one arm

It is obvious that the patient could not perform a breast stroke or crawl stroke, so the life-saving back stroke, without the use of the arms, is taught first. When the patient is able to travel a little way in comfort, sculling is introduced. Keeping the arms in the water, proceed now to teach the lateral arm stroke, a simple movement performed as follows:

1. The palms of the hands are drawn upwards along the thighs to reach the level of the hips, elbows bent sideways, to coincide with the bending of the knees.

2. The forearms are now extended sideways in line with the upper arms, the straight arms now being at an approximate angle of 30° to the trunk and coinciding with the sideways extension of the legs (*see* Fig. 2 (*a*)).

3. Keeping the arms and legs straight, pull the arms to the sides and bring the legs together, so that all limbs return at the same time to the starting position. The timing is easy to remember because arms and legs are performing similar movements:

When the knees are bent, the elbows are bent;
When the legs extend sideways, the arms extend sideways;
When the legs are brought together, the arms pull to the sides.

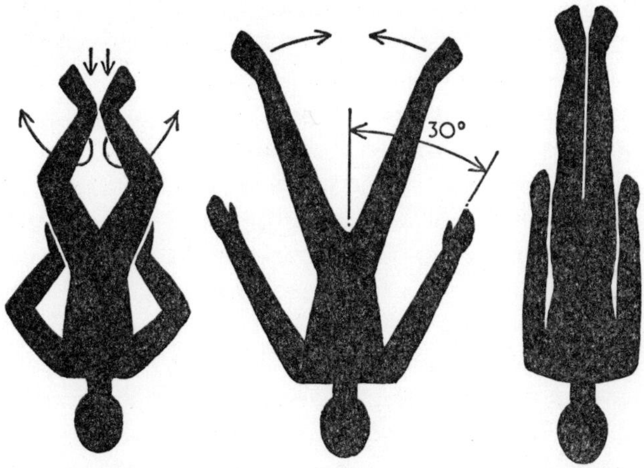

2 (*a*). The life-saving back stroke, for patients with weakness of one arm, showing the arms extended at an angle of 30°

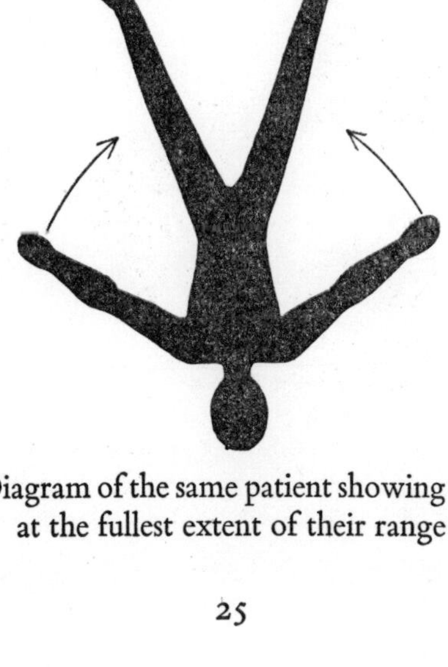

2 (*b*). Diagram of the same patient showing the arms at the fullest extent of their range

With practice, the arms (governed by the affected side) can be taken to the fullest extent of their range (*see* Fig. 2 (*b*)).

The next step is to teach the surface arm back stroke referred to and described on page 47, which when accomplished will give full range to the arms, still supported by the water. As the arms become stronger the breast stroke can be taught, but it is advisable not to teach either of the crawl strokes until the arm is strong enough to bear its own weight out of the water.

When there has been a weakness in one arm, I have noticed with a few pupils that when trying to swim the surface arm back stroke and the breast stroke, difficulty was encountered in extending the arms. The following method was adopted in both strokes with excellent results. When the arms are in the 'bent' position, the patient grasps the forefingers of the weak hand with the opposite hand and carries them forward to the extended position (*see* Fig. 3). When this is managed with ease, the patient places the fingers of the weak hand *on* to the opposite hand, and again the hands are carried forward to the

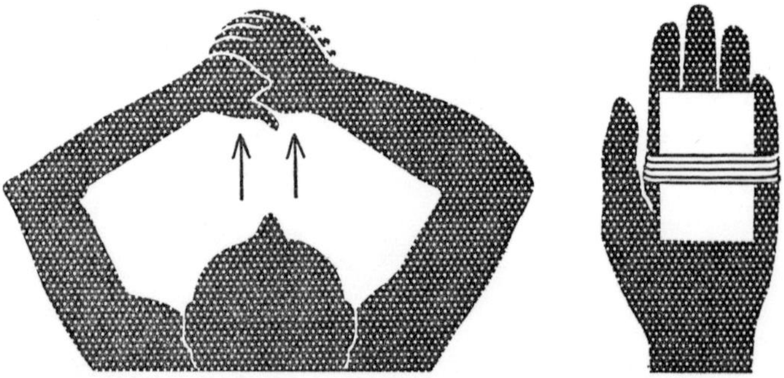

3. The breast stroke for a patient with weakness of one arm. The patient moves the weak hand to the extended position. A small piece of wood, held in the palm, keeps the weak fingers straight to obtain more power

extended position. With continued progress, the patient now feels that he is beginning to extend his arm, the weak one moving from the 'bent' position under its own power. The last stage is for the sound hand to flick the fingers of the weak hand and the arms will travel to the extended position. Where weakness in the fingers has been prevalent, resort was made to the use of a small piece of wood measuring approximately 3 in. by 2 in. by ¼ in. This is held in the palm of the hand, sometimes kept in place with a rubber band. Using this, the patient has to exert more power to overcome the resistance of the water, so that the extensor muscles benefit and become stronger.

Weakness of one side of the body

The life-saving back stroke is taught first, the method followed being that already described for an arm weakness.

The leg movements are taught in the ordinary way, and again range of movement, both with arms and legs, is governed by the degree of weakness. Before attempting the breast stroke, the patient should be able to swim a reasonable back stroke with the arms moving in a lateral direction. There is a weakness of the leg that may be encountered, so I refer to it along with a method which was adopted in two cases and which proved remarkably effective, but I must warn that there is no definite guarantee for its success in every case. Without a caliper the patient cannot walk, though he will eventually swim and, when in the water, the extensor muscles are so weak that he is unable to place his foot on the floor of the pool, as the buoyancy of the water lifts the leg at right angles to the thigh. The only way that the foot could be kept on the floor was by applying pressure with the hand on the knee.

A splint was tied on each side of the leg to keep the leg straight. To get accustomed to this the patient stood at shoulder level in the water with his back to the wall, without any ring support of any kind, his foot now on the floor of the pool. While I stood in front of him, he placed his hands on mine and followed as I walked backwards a few paces so that he obtained a 'stiff' leg sensation (*see* Fig. 4). The life-saving back stroke was taught while he still wore the splints, and both legs were kept perfectly straight.

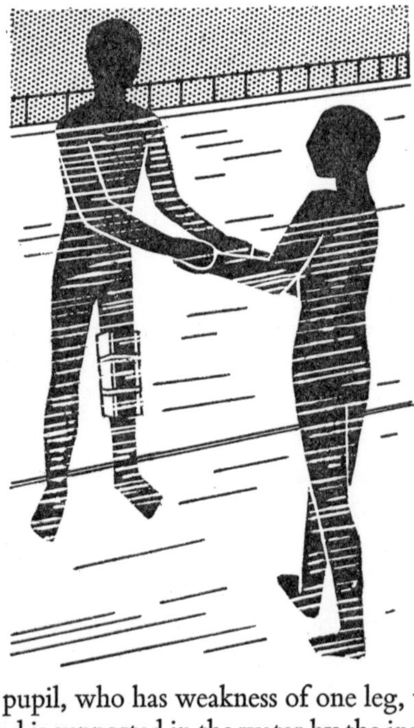

4. The pupil, who has weakness of one leg, wears a splint and is supported in the water by the instructor

By opening and closing his legs he got propulsion, and learned gradually that by bringing the legs together with more power his propulsion increased and gave him the feeling of stretching with his leg. After continued practice with the splints both in swimming and walking, we tried swimming without the splints. The result was very gratifying. He swam the stroke in the orthodox way, but the leg extension was now noticeable. When standing in the water, the foot did not rise to the original extent, and both swimming and walking improved correspondingly. Persevering on these lines, progress was marked chiefly by the improvement when walking. As the foot was being extended towards the floor of the pool he would assist with his hand by pushing the knee rather than by pressing and his foot would touch the floor.

With progressive improvement the push was made with the tips of the fingers, until assistance was no longer necessary and he then proceeded to learn the breast stroke. Eventually the leg regained strength and the caliper was discarded, although there was evidence of a limp when walking.

Weakness of both legs

As the body will balance more easily in the supine position, the life-saving back stroke with sculling is taught first, followed by the arms, in the water, moving in a lateral direction.

When the patient can swim with some proficiency and in comfort, it is possible to teach the breast stroke. Other strokes are complimentary.

Weakness of neck muscles

In order to mobilize and strengthen the neck muscles, the theme of instruction is directed towards the performance of forward and backward somersaults in the 'tuck' position which, when correctly executed, has the shoulders square to the water (*see* Fig. 5). The head is educated in helping to balance the body and maintain its position.

Forward and backward gliding should be taught, ensuring that the pupil steers a straight course. Proceed to teach the breast stroke and the life-saving back stroke and then surface diving, to be followed by both forward and backward somersaults. Other strokes are complimentary and, when teaching the front crawl, it is most essential that the correct breathing technique is mastered and that the head does not return to an abnormal position.

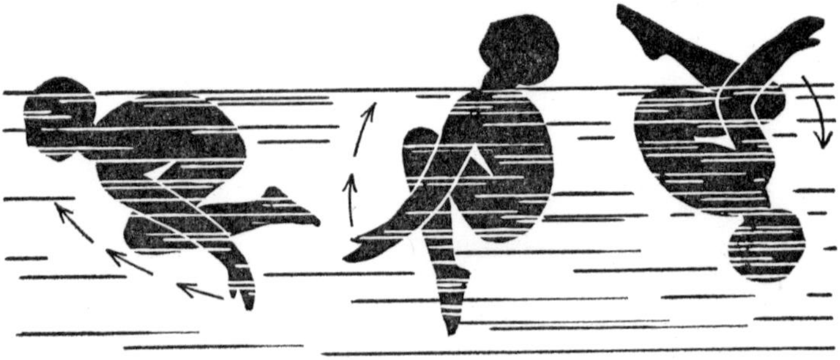

5. Backward somersaults in the 'tuck' position help to strengthen weak neck muscles

Progress can be measured by the following skills:

Executing, without pause, two forward somersaults followed by two backward ones. Swimming three strokes, then making a surface dive and repeating this to the end of the pool. Swimming the length or width of the pool, depending, of course, on the pupil's ability; with, at first, breathing in, unilaterally, the first swim should be done on the left side, the second swim on the right side and for the third swim the head is turned alternately to the left and right side when breathing in.

Chapter III

DISABILITIES DUE TO PHYSICAL DEFECT

Spinal disabilities

These are kyphosis or 'round back', lordosis or 'hollow back' and scoliosis or lateral curve of the spine.

The spine determines the posture of the body, and as the weight of the spine is transmitted to the legs through the medium of the pelvis it is essential, particularly to the growing child, to develop good strong muscles round the pelvic girdle. A breast stroke leg action is, I believe, better suited to achieve this than the crawl, as there is a wider range of movement in comparison with the close up and down action of the crawl strokes. To teach a person suffering from any of the complaints listed above the obvious choice would seem to be the breast stroke. It is, of course, imperative to choose a stroke where the limbs on both sides are working together, performing the same movements at the same time and *not* to teach an asymmetrical crawl stroke. A better choice than the breast stroke is the surface arm back stroke, as it is almost identical with the breast stroke and has the added advantage that the water is taking the weight of the spine better in this supine position, so that breathing is easy to control and balance is easier to maintain. The life-saving back stroke kick is taught first with arms sculling and then with the arms moving in a lateral direction, and then proceeding with the surface arm movement.

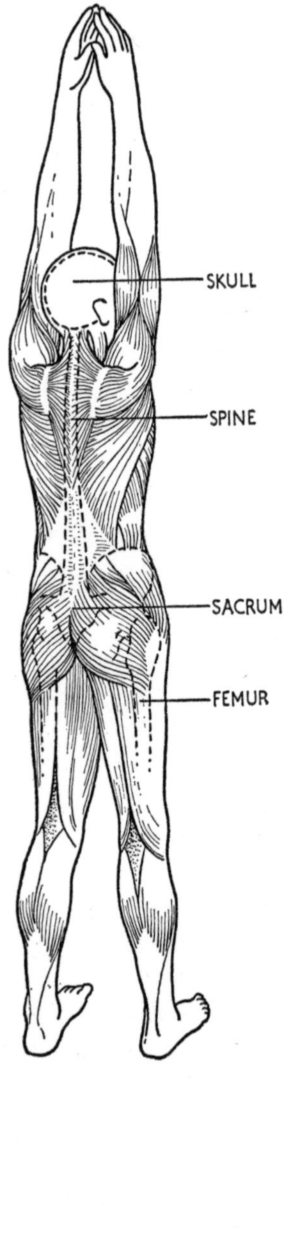

6. Diagram showing the position of the muscles and the bones when the body is held fully stretched with the arms, trunk and legs in a straight line

This stroke enables both the long and the short muscles of the spine to benefit and to coax the spine back to a natural position. The long spinal muscles extend from the sacrum to the base of the skull and are so arranged as to distribute a pull over the widest possible area to allow movement of extension at different levels of the spine (*see* Fig. 6).

In order that the intended benefit of straightening the spine may be obtained, the body should be held for an appreciable time in the correct full-stretch position, with arms, trunk and legs in a straight line, legs together, arms together, head resting naturally on the water, and eyes directed towards the roof.

The thorax also benefits. As the arms are extended beyond the head the cavity of the thorax is lengthened and broadened as the arms sweep outwards and sideways to regain the starting position, allowing more room for the lungs to expand. A person who floats naturally will be able to hold this pose indefinitely, while a non-floater has to rely on momentum to help in maintaining balance. Should difficulties arise, a good alternative is to tuck the feet under the rail with a ring support at the hips, and perform the exercise using the arms only (*see* Fig. 7). Jerking or pushing the arms vigorously beyond the

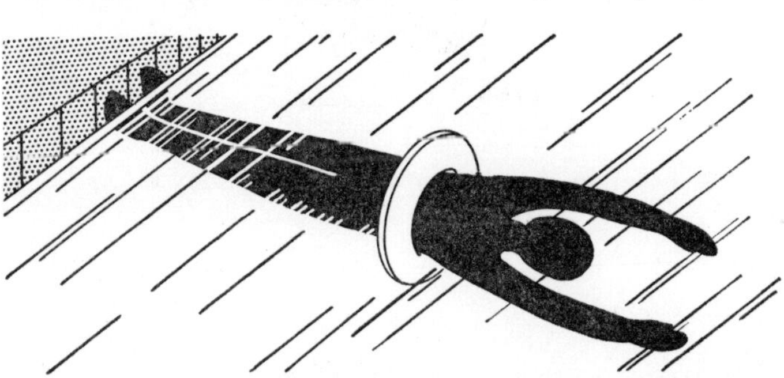

7. A patient with a spinal disability floating with arms extended, feet under the rail and a ring support at the hips

head should be avoided. It is better to slide the arms easily to the fullest extent.

Flat feet

This is caused by the flattening of the longitudinal or plantar arch. When the foot is actively stretched, i.e. bent downward away from the knee in plantar flexion, it is extended as the tibial muscles elevate the plantar arch to a more normal and natural state. Any swimming stroke is beneficial as a corrective exercise, the very action of the feet producing plantar flexion and this can be observed during the down beat of the legs in the back crawl and the upward thrust in the front crawl and during the sweep of the legs in the breast and life-saving back strokes (*see* Fig. 8).

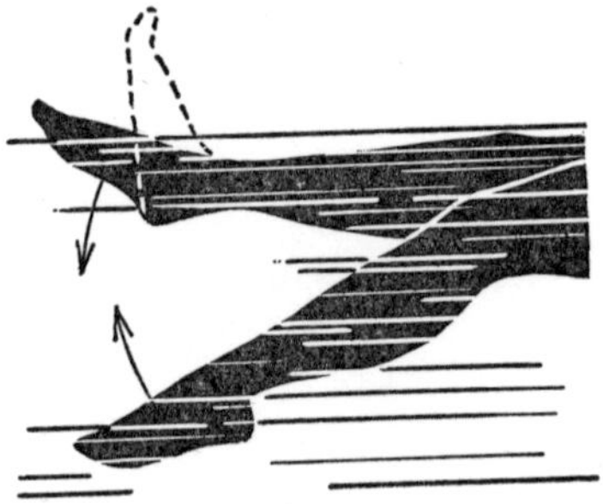

8. Diagram showing how swimming encourages plantar flexion

Talipes

These patients, having a concentration of bone, with hardly any flexibility of the ankles, find the crawl strokes at first somewhat arduous to learn. This type of pupil responds better to the breast stroke, and eventually becomes very adept and strong at life-saving. When learning the crawl, the use of flippers is found to be of great advantage, as these convey to him the sense of flexibility and of the undulating motion of the leg action.

It takes some time, however, for these pupils to swim a reasonable crawl stroke in comfort. As an outdoor exercise, cycling is beneficial.

Loss of one arm

A person who has suffered the loss of an arm or leg is at the outset unequally balanced, and for the purpose of illustration we shall assume that the amputation has been of the left arm.

Forward and backward gliding are taught first. Naturally during the initial stages the body will incline somewhat towards the right hand side, due to the extra weight on that side.

By keeping the legs straight and close together and at the same time depressing the left shoulder, a sufficient balance will be attained to perform a respectable glide.

Instructions

1. Proceed now to teach both the life-saving back stroke (without using the arms) and the back crawl leg kick.

2. Use a rubber ring support, and if the body is unevenly balanced reach over, towards the left side, to grasp the ring with the right hand to counteract the imbalance (*see* Fig. 9). When the ring support is dispensed with, place the right hand across the body to maintain balance, until the patient is able to keep his balance by pressure of the left shoulder.

3. Introduce now the back crawl arm stroke, and with a little practice, even with one arm only, the patient will swim a straight course. He will experience a lot of frustration and

some difficulty when trying to swim in a prone position or on the side and will find greater comfort on the back.

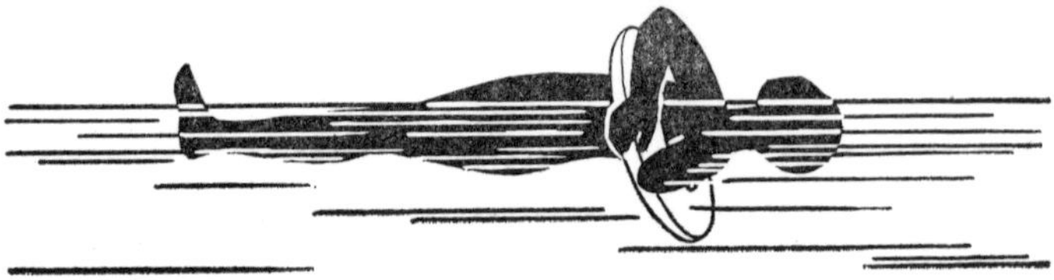

9. A one-armed patient, wearing a rubber ring under the arm-pits for the life-saving back stroke. The right hand reaches over the body to hold the ring and correct the imbalance

Loss of one leg

Let us assume that the left leg has been amputated.

The front glide should be taught first. The body will naturally incline towards the right side but this can be corrected by depressing the left shoulder and exerting a little pressure with the left arm to restore balance.

Instructions

Proceed to teach the side stroke, with the patient lying on the right side, recovering the left arm along the surface of the water and directing the eyes well towards the left shoulder so that the head is well positioned to maintain the sideways balance. This type of stroke will be found to be best suited to a patient with this particular disability.

Loss of both legs

A person who has suffered the loss of both legs is 'unsinkable' and can immediately propel himself by lying on his back and either sculling or using a lateral movement of the arms. In the prone position he can cultivate a side stroke and an alternative over-arm stroke with bi-lateral breathing.

Chapter IV

GENERAL DISABILITIES

Blindness

The blind are usually very good pupils, as they are full of concentration. They do not suffer the usual distractions and together with that sixth sense which they seem to develop, they have an uncanny knack of applying themselves.

When a blind person first enters the building he is immediately aware of being in a strange environment. Before proceeding to the pool, he should be met in the hall of the building so that the teacher and pupil may become closely associated through a friendly chat. The teacher should explain the layout of the building, the strange odour of chlorine that permeates it, the noise and sound of splashing, etc., and in general make the pupil as familiar with the local atmosphere as a sighted person would be.

Instructions

1. On entering the pool, describe its construction, appointments, etc., and take the pupil to a cubicle. If possible, use the same one for each visit, so that the pupil becomes familiar with the positions of seat, clothes' hooks, curtain, etc. When he is prepared for the water, escort him to the toilet and foot bath.

2. Before proceeding with the lesson, sit down and explain one or two details relating to density, relaxation and so on, which will help him to understand and co-operate in subsequent exercises.

3. Lead him by the hand down the steps of the pool, telling him how many steps he has to negotiate, and inform him when his foot is about to touch the water. When his arm is level with the parapet, get him to place his hand upon it and as he descends the steps he will be able to judge the depth and find his bearings. With his hand now on the rail, guide him along to the deeper water which he will gauge by the level of his chest.

4. Holding his hands, let him submerge until his chin is touching the surface of the water. Remember that he has to learn to judge distance by touch, so repeat this several times, but be very watchful that no water enters his mouth.

5. Eventually, still holding his hands, get him to bob up and down, so that he can gauge when his chin is touching the water. Walk with him across the pool and he will come to realize the weight and pressure of the water and also to assess the width of the pool.

6. With his hands supported by the rail, the pupil is taught 'bubble' blowing; he then repeats this using the teacher's hands for support and finally does it alone.

7. Prepare to teach the life-saving back stroke, as in this the pupil has only the leg movement to concentrate on and breathing is easy and unimpaired. In the initial stages use a rubber ring support. Let him lie on his back, toes tucked under the rail, head supported by the teacher, and get him to breathe and relax. Teach him to push and glide, later add sculling and then let him repeat this without using the ring support.

To teach the leg action, the pupil adopts the *prone* position and holds the rail, with the teacher guiding the legs in the breast stroke kick (*see* Fig. 10 (*a*)). Later, with the teacher supporting him under the chest, the pupil performs the leg action until he has properly acquired it and eventually repeats it without the teacher's support.

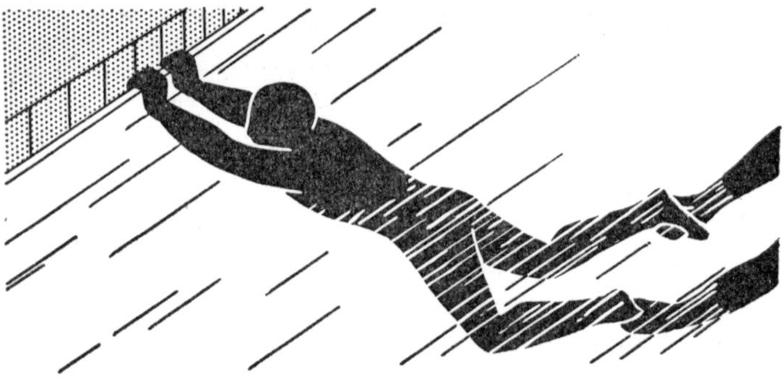

10 (*a*). A blind pupil, learning the leg action of the life-saving back stroke. The prone position is adopted while the teacher guides his legs

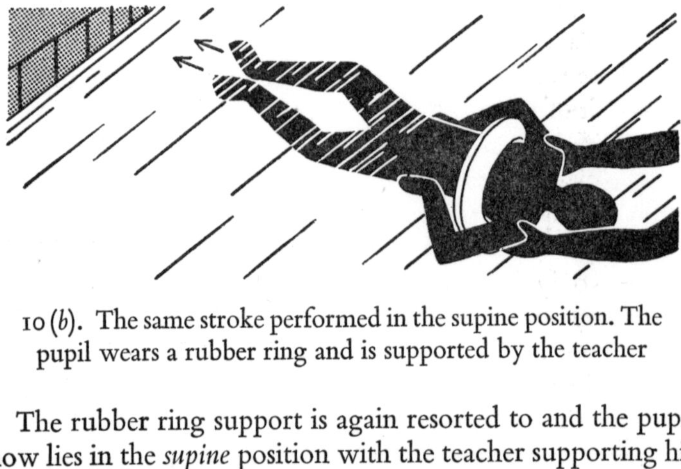

10 (*b*). The same stroke performed in the supine position. The pupil wears a rubber ring and is supported by the teacher

The rubber ring support is again resorted to and the pupil now lies in the *supine* position with the teacher supporting his head or the shoulders (*see* Fig. 10 (*b*)). He performs the breast stroke kick already acquired and which is later adjusted to the correct back stroke kick with lower legs dropping etc. Sculling is then introduced. This is continued in a similar manner without the ring support and eventually without the teacher's support for the head. The pupil is encouraged to swim with

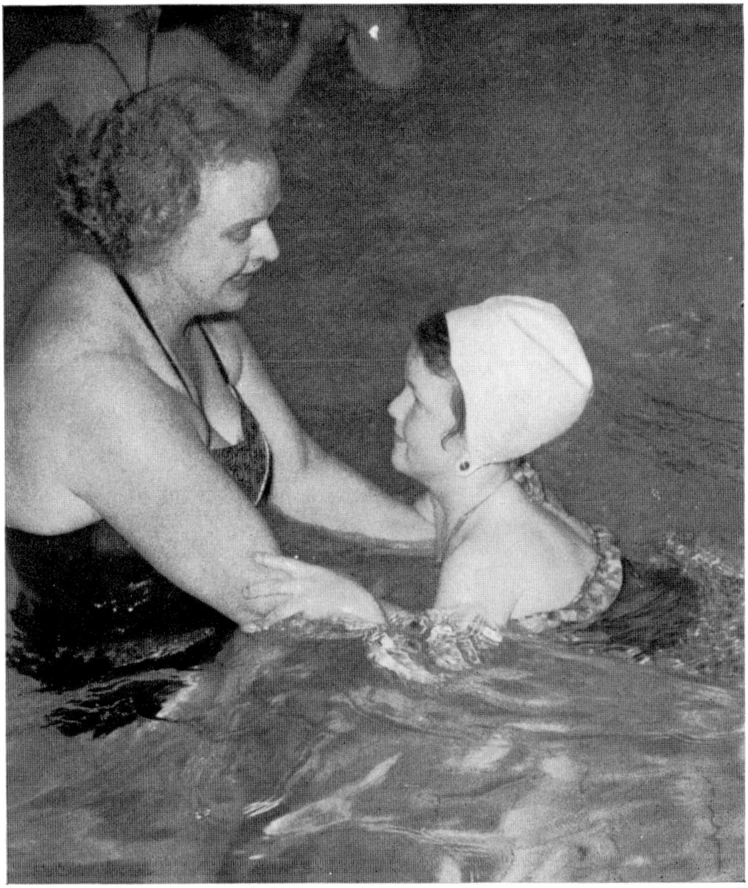

I. The wife of the author, formerly Miss 'Sunny' Lowry, an English Channel swimmer, gives individual help whilst teaching a group of spastic and paralysed children

(*a*)

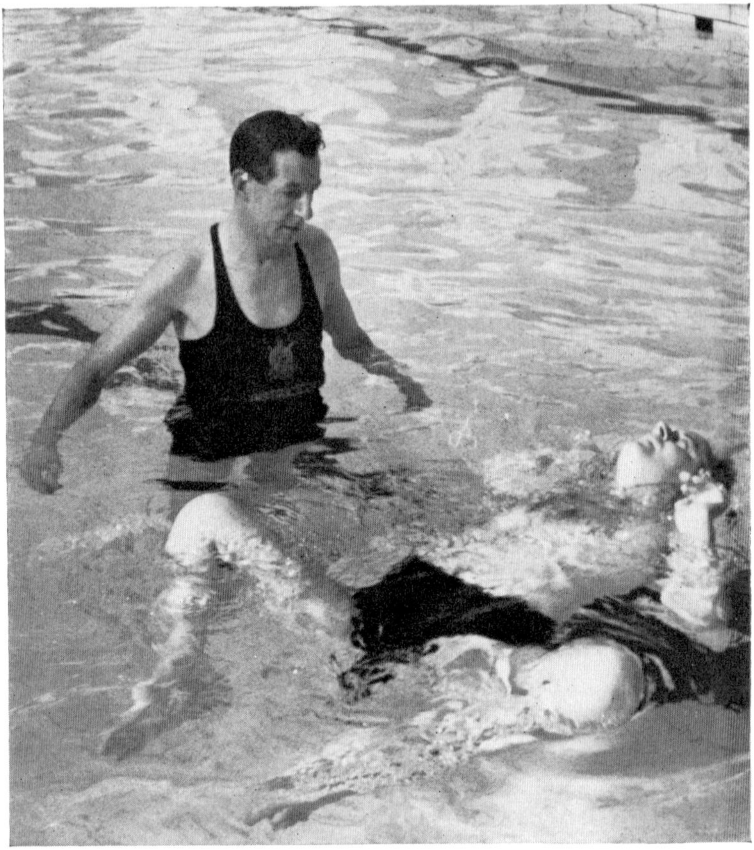

II (*a*), (*b*) and (*c*). Three positions of the surface arm back stroke. This pupil had paralysis of both legs and the left arm and is being taught by the author (*see p. 47*)

(b)

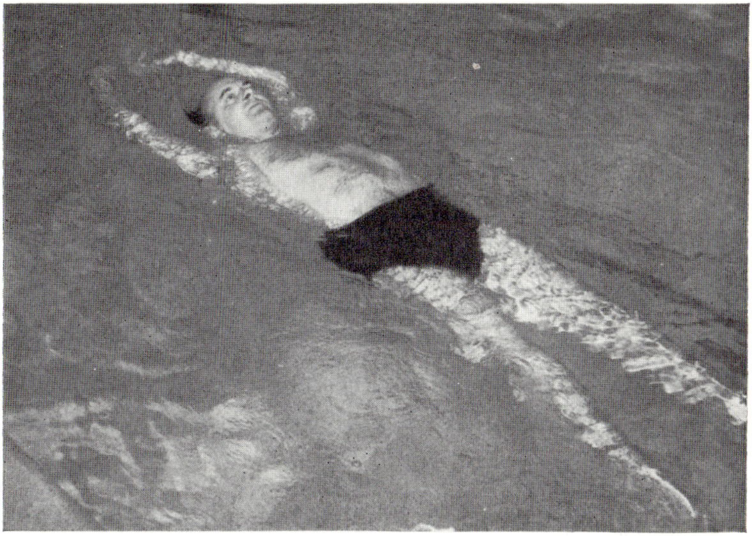

(c)

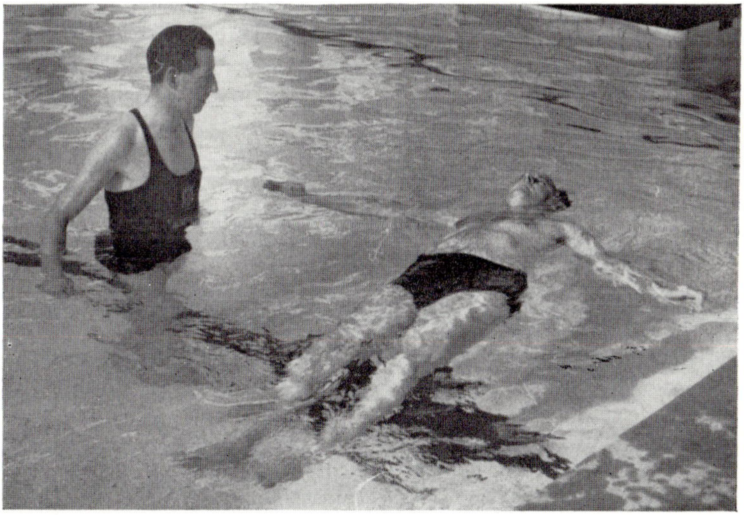

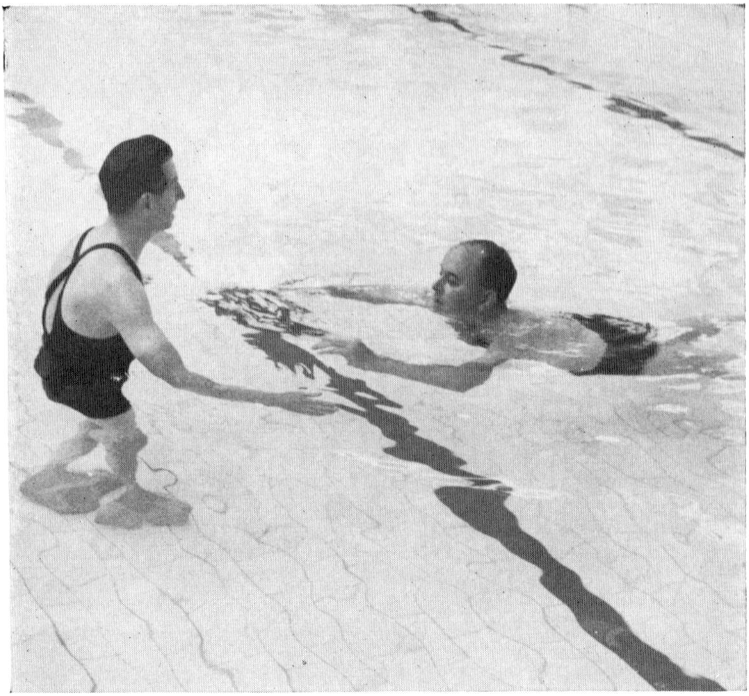

III. The same pupil as in Plate II is helped by the author to master the breast stroke. Notice the disturbance of the water in the region of the right hand. The left arm is not strong enough to press downward to assist in stabilizing the body. Consequently the balance of the body is upset and in an effort to effect its recovery the right hand has 'feathered' close to the surface of the water (*see p. 49*)

his hands on his hips to cultivate a stronger kick. At this stage the breast stroke can be introduced.

The leg action will have already been mastered, so the teacher now progresses with forward gliding exercises and then on to the arm stroke. The teacher stands in the water behind the pupil, grasps his arms and guides them through the exercise until the pupil is familiar with the exercise and can perform it alone. With the ring support, he now swims the complete stroke and eventually the support is discarded altogether.

When swimming the width or length of the pool, the pupil should count the number of strokes he uses, in order that he is able to measure his distance. As he becomes adept at both these strokes the crawl strokes can be proceeded with, the teacher operating the legs and arms in the initial stages.

It will for a while be found necessary for the teacher to guide the pupil to swim in a straight line. This can be done from the side of the pool with such directions as 'pull a little with the right', etc.

Other skills can then be introduced such as floating and surface diving. When he is proficient at surface diving the pupil can be taught to dive, with the teacher always notifying him of the height of the parapet from the water, so that he can judge his entry accordingly. As he is unable to register the results of his efforts by seeing, it is encouraging to introduce him to the regular bathers who no doubt will have observed his progress. He will enjoy swimming alongside them and no doubt they will bestow some very helpful and complimentary praise.

Deaf and dumb pupils

People thus afflicted are not dumb in the accepted sense, but having never been able to hear or recognize sounds, they are as a natural consequence unable to repeat them and so become inarticulate. It is pleasing and gratifying to note that speech therapy has made a tremendous advance in this field and is playing a major part in assisting those whom I prefer to regard as inarticulate.

In passing it is gratifying also to note that during the course of swimming lessons I have heard these people begin to make audible and recognizable sounds. As with the blind, I find the deaf to be good subjects for tuition, as they must concentrate on the teacher for lip reading and instructional signs.

Presuming that exercises aimed at acquiring confidence and learning the correct breathing, by blowing bubbles, etc., have been completed, I adopt the following method in teaching the deaf to swim.

Instructions

1. Gliding is taught first. The teacher demonstrates each position of the arms, legs, head and so on, and performs the glide. The pupil follows and corrections are made by the teacher accordingly.

2. Proceed to the breast stroke leg movements. Here I enlist the help of an assistant.

   (*a*) The assistant grasps the rail in the position for the leg stroke drill. The teacher takes the assistant's legs and guides them in detail through the drill, while the pupil watches and is encouraged to 'repeat after me', that is, to imitate the teacher's instructions with his lips when saying 'bend', 'out wide', 'together straight'.

   (*b*) Next the teacher grasps the rail himself, his legs being guided by the *pupil*, with the assistant encouraging the pupil to 'mouth the movements'.

(*c*) The pupil now grasps the rail and is guided by the teacher.

(*d*) The assistant grasps the rail, supported by the teacher under the chest and performs the leg drill.

(*e*) The teacher is supported by the pupil and repeats (*d*).

(*f*) The pupil is supported by the teacher and repeats (*d*).

(*g*) The assistant grasps the rail and unsupported performs the leg drill.

(*h*) The teacher grasps the rail and unsupported repeats (*g*).

(*i*) The pupil grasps the rail and unsupported repeats (*g*).

This method of repetition enables the pupil to gain a good and accurate picture of what is required and since it is so helpful it is desirable, as he progresses to other strokes, to enlist the aid of an assistant in a similar way when demonstrating leg exercises on the rail.

3. The teacher now demonstrates the use of the 'kicking board' (*see* Fig. 11) and, with the aid of a rubber ring support, the pupil repeats the teacher's movements, ultimately dispensing with the ring support.

4. The arm stroke is now taught.

(*a*) Standing with his shoulders in the water, the teacher demonstrates the arm movement.

(*b*) The teacher now stands behind the pupil, takes his arms and guides them through the drill.

(*c*) With the teacher standing in front of and facing the pupil, both now perform the drill, the teacher's movements being 'mirrored' by the pupil, who is again encouraged to 'press', 'bend', 'stretch', etc., all the time repeating the words with his lips. *Note:* The teacher must check that the breathing sequence is timed correctly.

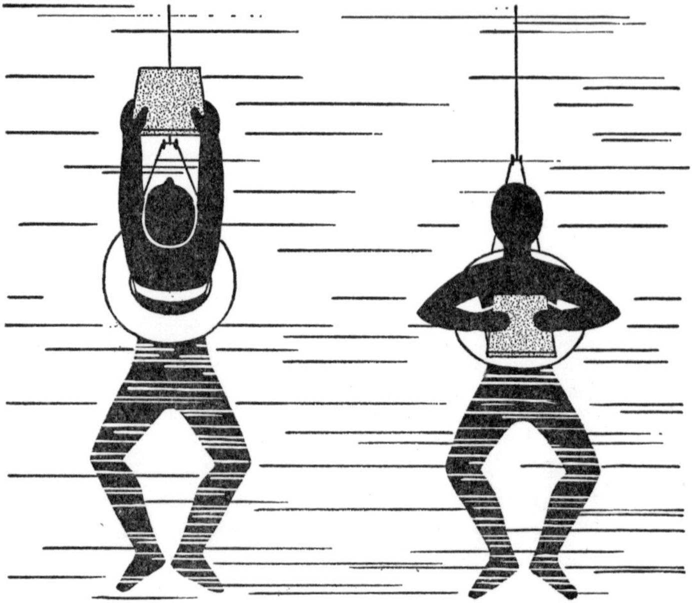

11. Use of the 'kicking board' in teaching the breast stroke leg action. In the prone position the arms are extended, in the supine position the board is clasped to the chest

(*d*) The teacher swims a demonstration of the full stroke.

(*e*) The pupil, with ring support, repeats (*d*), progressing until the support can be discarded.

Other strokes can be taught in a similar way and, when giving instruction in diving and life-saving, an assistant is most desirable and helpful.

Chapter V

SWIMMING STROKES

There is a wide selection of textbooks from which to choose and learn the finer techniques involved in the various strokes. It is opportune to refer to the strokes here and to describe them in broad outline as a basis with which to begin. It is advisable to note that the life-saving back stroke, as well as the life-saving back stroke with lateral arm movement, the surface arm back stroke, and the breast stroke are all symmetrical strokes. The back and front crawl strokes, however, are anti-symmetrical and must not be taught to a person suffering from infantile paralysis.

The life-saving back stroke

In the life-saving back stroke the legs only are used in a similar way to that of the breast stroke, except that here the rule to remember is that the knees must not come above the surface and if this is observed the stroke becomes comparatively easy to swim.

Position ready. Lie on the back, the head resting naturally and comfortably on the water, the hands resting on the hips, or with the arms folded across the chest, the legs extended and together.

1. Bend the knees allowing the feet to drop downwards until the legs are at right angles to the thighs while the knees open until they are approximately 6 in. apart.

2. The legs swing outwards and in a strong circular sweep

are brought upwards and together to the extended position in preparation for the next stroke.

Note. Throughout the movement the thighs should be in line with the body, just below the surface of the water, and care should be taken to avoid a sitting position. The lowering of the legs should be slow and effortless, while the outward and upward swing which provides propulsion should be strong and steady. A short glide with the legs together between each stroke is restful.

The life-saving back stroke with arms moving laterally

Position ready. Lie on the back, legs straight and together, arms by the sides and head resting comfortably on the water.

1. *Legs.* The legs are used in exactly the same manner already described in the life-saving back stroke.

2. *Arms and legs.* As the legs are lowered into the water, slide the palms of the hands upwards along the thighs until the fingers reach the hips, keeping the arms just below the surface of the water. The arms and legs bend simultaneously.

3. The arms and legs are now straightened and extended sideways, with all limbs extending simultaneously.

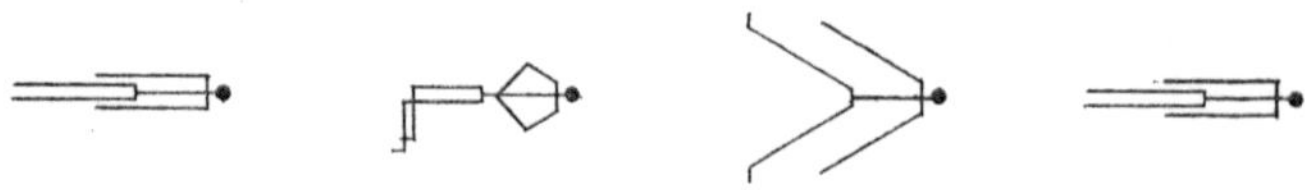

Position 'Ready'

1. Arms and legs bend simultaneously

2. Arms and legs extend sideways simultaneously

3. Arms and legs brought together simultaneously to position 'Ready'

12. The life-saving back stroke—with arms moving laterally

4. Keeping the legs straight, they are now brought together for propulsion and are assisted by the arms, which at the same time are kept straight and brought to the sides in preparation for the next stroke. A short glide between each stroke will be restful. At all times the arms and legs work simultaneously (*see* Fig. 12).

The surface arm back stroke

Position ready. Lie on the back with the legs straight and together, arms by the sides, palms inwards, head resting comfortably on the water.

As the legs work exactly as already described in the life-saving back stroke, a description of the arm movements working in conjunction with the legs is given.

1. *Arms*. Keep the arms close to the sides just below the surface of the water. Turn the palms of the hands to face downwards, thumbs and forefingers touching the thighs. Still touching the sides of the thighs, bend the elbows sideways, drawing the hands upwards and keeping the fingernails behind the seam of the costume, until the backs of the fingertips, the nails, touch the top of the head and behind the ears, the thumbs uppermost. This keeps the arms square to the water and prevents water splashing on to the face. As the arms are carrying out this movement, the legs are lowered into the water, so that the arms and legs bend simultaneously.

2. In this position, turn the palms of the hands uppermost and at the same time begin to straighten the arms and extend them beyond the head with the hands together. As the arms are carrying out this movement, the legs begin to straighten and extend sideways.

3. The arms continue to straighten until they reach their fullest extent and at the same time the legs are kept straight

and brought together, so that the whole body is now in a full gliding position, the bringing together of the legs coinciding with the full stretch of the arms. When this position is reached, glide and rest.

At the end of the glide, keeping the legs still, the arms are now swept outwards and downwards to resume the 'ready' position in preparation for the next stroke (*see* Fig. 13).

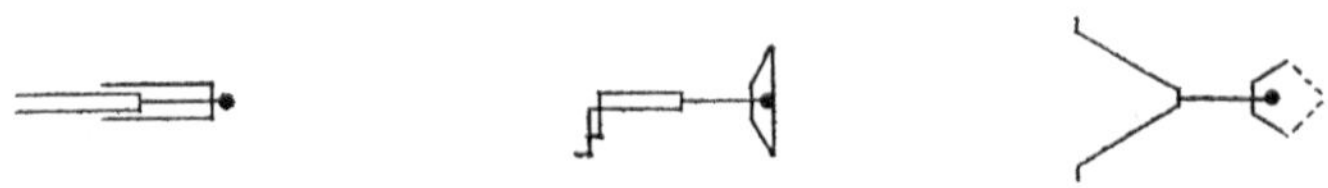

Position 'Ready'

1. Arms and legs bend simultaneously

2. Legs extend sideways as the arms are moving into the Full Stretch position

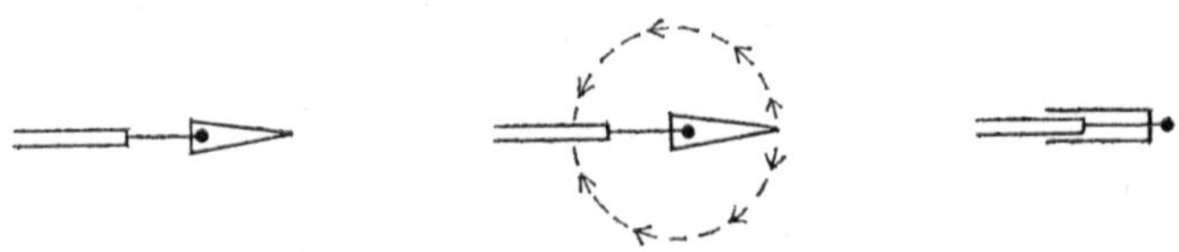

3. The legs are brought together to coincide with the full stretch of the arms. Note. GLIDE in this position

4. At the end of the glide, keeping the legs still, the arms are swept OUTWARDS and DOWNWARDS to the resumed position 'Ready'

5. Position 'Ready'

13. The surface arm back stroke

Note. It is most essential to get the timing of the arms and legs correct, i.e. when the arms are bent, the legs are bent, etc.

I personally consider this to be the finest remedial stroke of all. All the limbs are supported by the water all the time, while breathing is easy and unrestricted. The respiratory organs and chest muscles are strengthened, and it affords a comfortable and pleasant way to swim for the 'not so young'.

The breast stroke

Position ready. Begin with a forward glide in the prone position with the arms extended, keeping the hands together, the legs extended with the feet together, shoulders in the water and the eyes looking straight ahead.

1. Keeping the arms straight, press them outwards and downwards, breathe in through the mouth and keep the legs still. This will give some slight propulsion though the main effect is to balance the body in preparation for the co-ordination of the legs.

2. Bend the arms, bringing the elbows to the chest, with the hands slightly in advance of the chin, the palms facing downwards and at the same time bend the knees outward, not under the body, keeping the heels together and drawing them towards the buttocks.

3. Keeping the hands together push them gently, not vigorously, forward to the extended position and at the same time breathe out through the nose and mouth. As the arms are executing this movement the legs now swing outwards and backwards in a circular movement until they reach the extended position with the legs straight and together in preparation for the next stroke. The legs should be brought together with some vigour as this is the chief propulsive movement of the stroke.

Note. Remember to keep the shoulders in the water and to inhale and exhale at the correct time with each cycle. This will induce relaxation which is most important and, as the learner becomes more proficient, he will exhale with his face in the water and on the completion of the stroke execute a glide which provides a useful rest.

The back crawl stroke

Position ready. Glide on the back, hands held loosely by the sides, the head resting comfortably on the water and look towards the toes with the hips slightly submerged. Avoid a sitting position.

1. *Legs*. Commence to move the legs up and down, and scull with the hands at the same time. The legs move continuously up and down so that at the top of each beat the toes, but not the heels, break the surface. The feet drop alternately to a depth of approximately 6–9 in., varying with different pupils. Hold the feet loosely and turn them slightly inwards. The whole movement is a loose whip-like one and should originate from the hips, while the knees and ankles should be flexible in order to bend against the resistance of the water. On no account must they be stiff.

2. *Arms*. With the palm outward lift the right arm clear of the water, keeping the arm straight, and swing it, loosely held, to a position in advance of and in line with the shoulder where the hand, little finger first, enters the water.

3. The arm now pulls with a circular sweep just beneath the surface towards the right thigh, during which time the left arm is recovered clear of the water, palm outwards, and swings over to the advanced position so that both arms are alternating.

Note. There is no hesitation in the movement of the arms. As soon as the pull has been completed, the arm is lifted clear of the water and recovered to the entry position in advance of the shoulder. As the face is clear of the water all the time, there is no restriction to breathing.

The front crawl stroke

Position ready. Forward glide.

1. *Legs*. As in the back crawl, the legs move alternately up and down, but at the top of each beat in the front crawl the heels, and not the toes, break the surface. Both in the front and back crawl strokes the legs are the chief agents in maintaining the balance of the body so good leg work is essential, and the dog paddle is recommended as an exercise to practise and develop a good leg movement.

2. *Dog paddle*. Keeping the head in a central position, the chin on the water, look forward, and as the legs move up and down, press the hands alternately downwards and backwards beneath the body one after the other, in a way similar to that in which a dog uses its front paws when swimming.

3. *Arms*. Once a satisfactory balance is established with a good rhythm of the legs, begin to lift the arms out of the water in recovery. The right hand enters the water in front of the shoulder in comfortable reach so that there is a gentle slope from the elbow down to the fingertips. The hand now presses down and back with the arm still slightly bent at the elbow until the hand reaches a position directly below the shoulder, when the arm is straightened and the hand continues its drive back to leave the water as the thumb brushes the thigh. The elbow is now bent sufficiently to lift the hand clear of the water, and the arm, which must be completely relaxed, is carried forward to the entry position with the hand entering the water in front of the shoulder. As the right arm begins its downward pull, the left arm begins its recovery so that both arms are working alternately without hesitation.

4. *Breathing*. Let us assume that the swimmer breathes on his right side. As the right elbow bends to recover the arm from the water, the head is turned, without being lifted, to the

right and a breath is taken in sharply through the mouth. As the arm is moving forward to the entry position, the head is turned back again to its central position with the face in the water and the breath is exhaled slowly.

Note. The stroke, which should be performed rhythmically and without pause, is composed of three rhythms all co-ordinated into one.

(*a*) The rhythm of the arms, chiefly for propulsion.
(*b*) The rhythm of the legs, chiefly for balance.
(*c*) The rhythm of the head, for breathing.

Correct breathing in any stroke is essential, as it induces relaxation. Unless a swimmer can breathe in comfort, he will not swim in comfort.

Muscle action related to swimming

The limbs are the levers of the body, operating in various ways according to the task performed and powered and guided by muscular activity.

When a limb is moved, a complex arrangement of muscles is involved. Some act as agonists, others as antagonists, while the fibres, according to their construction, can influence the direction and action of a limb. The middle fibres of the deltoid, for instance, abduct or lift the arms sideways to approximately a horizontal position. The anterior fibres perform flexion of the upper arms by drawing them up to a vertical position above the head, while the posterior fibres draw the upper arms backward in extension. Muscles, therefore, are inter-related and work in groups.

It is well to consider here the abdominal muscles which are so very important to the structure of the body. They not only act as a protection for the viscera, they also assist in respiration, in movement, and, like the spine, influence the posture of the

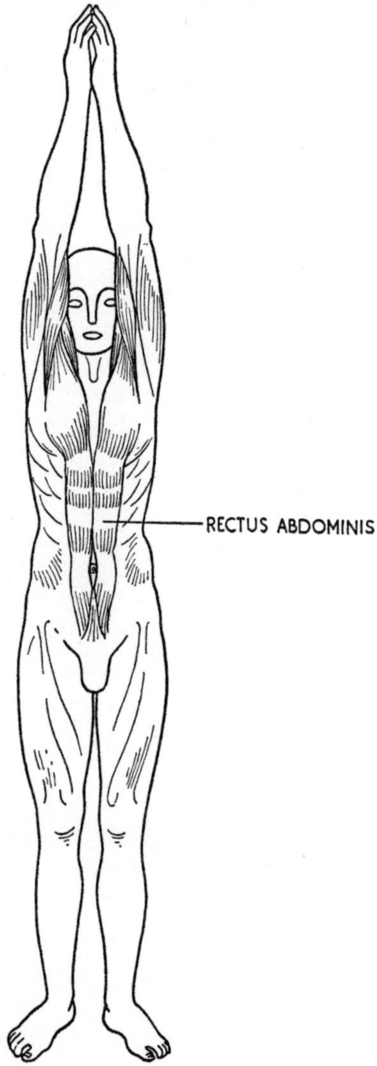

14. Diagram showing the rectus abdominis muscles

body. A good firm abdominal wall is, therefore, extremely desirable.

When swimming, the abdominal wall has a steadying effect upon the trunk, which must remain passive, correctly and easily balanced, to be transported through the water by the limbs. The abdominal wall, then, can be regarded as the platform between the lower limbs and the shoulders, allowing free mobility of the limbs (*see* Fig. 14). Great benefit can, therefore, be derived from abdominal and dorsal exercises.

Chapter VI

SUGGESTED EXERCISES

These should be carried out in the pool, with the body and limbs immersed as much as possible.

The neck

Position. Standing.
Exercise. (*a*) Bend neck forward.
(*b*) Bend neck backward.
(*c*) Bend neck sideways.
(*d*) Turn head sideways, to the left and right alternately.
(*e*) Rotate head to the left and right alternately.

Hip abductors and adductors

Position. Stand facing and holding the rail, with the legs together.
Exercise. (*a*) Make a slight jump, straddling the legs sideways.
(*b*) Close legs together.
(*c*) Cross legs.
(*d*) Bring legs together to starting position.

Hip flexors and extensors

Position. Float vertically, with a rubber ring support under the arm-pits.

Exercise. Keeping the knees straight, move the legs backward and forward in a scissors movement. Both legs must work together; as one is moving forward, the other must be moving backward.

Knee flexors and extensors

Exercise No. 1

Position. Standing, with the legs together.

(*a*) Bend the right knee, holding the calf at right angles to the thigh.

(*b*) Straighten the leg and return it to the starting position.

(*c*) Repeat the exercise with the left leg.

Exercise No. 2

Position. Using a rubber ring support, lie on the back, with the legs straight and together.

(*a*) Bend the right knee, letting the foot sink down into the water, with the calf at right angles to the thigh.

(*b*) Straighten the leg and return it to the starting position.

(*c*) Repeat with the left leg.

In Exercise No. 1 the flexors are assisted by buoyancy, and the extensors are resisted by buoyancy.

In Exercise No. 2 the flexors are resisted by buoyancy, and the extensors are assisted by buoyancy.

Note. When performing these exercises, care should be taken to keep the thighs together.

Spinal exercises

FOR KYPHOSIS

Position. Standing, with the feet astride.

Exercise. Raise the arms sideways, turning the palms upwards; stretch the arms backwards, pressing the head backwards with the chin well in.

For Lordosis

Position. Standing, with the back to the wall and the arms by the sides.

Exercise. Press the hollow of the back to the wall; then relax. Repeat.

For Scoliosis

Position. Standing, with the legs astride and the hips firm.

Exercise. (*a*) Bend the trunk from side to side.
(*b*) Turn the trunk slowly to the left side to make a full turn.
(*c*) Repeat to the right side.

Arms and shoulders

Exercise No. 1

Position. Stand with the arms close to the sides, and bend the elbows upwards.

Stretch the arms forwards, sideways, upwards and downwards.

Exercise No. 2

Position. Stand with the hands over-grasping the rail support.

Walk the arms sideways, hand over hand along the rail, with the legs still and hanging loosely.

Combined shoulder and elbow exercise

Position. Face the wall and over-grasp the rail, placing the feet on the wall.

Exercise. (*a*) Bend the elbows, drawing the chest towards the wall and keeping the legs still.
(*b*) Straighten the elbows, pushing the chest away from the wall.

Forearms

Position. Standing or sitting, with the arms close to the sides and the elbows bent.

Exercise. Pronate and supinate the forearms.

If a stick approximately 6 in. long is held in each hand, progress can be measured by aligning the sticks as near to the vertical as possible.

Feet and ankles

Exercise. (*a*) Pick up small objects, marbles, etc., with the toes.
(*b*) Raise and lower the heels.
(*c*) Walk.
(*d*) Walk on tiptoes.
(*e*) Hop from side to side with the knees slightly bent.
(*f*) With the use of a 'kicking board' perform crawl and breast stroke leg exercises.

Weak fingers and hands

Exercise. Grasp a small rubber sponge in each hand.
(*a*) Immerse the sponges in the water.
(*b*) Raise them clear of the water and squeeze them dry. Progress can be measured by 'dryness'.

Chapter VII

GROUP TEACHING

Group teaching can be carried out with every success, provided that certain safeguards, recommended below, are observed.

Composition of the group

The group should be composed of a director to take charge; a team of adult assistants (swimmers) who are prepared to attend each session with faithful regularity, in order that they can become familiar with, and appreciate the theme of instruction. The pupils should not be confined to one particular disability and should number approximately ten as a comfortable working unit. The director, in charge of operations, should be a doctor or physiotherapist with a knowledge of swimming strokes, or a professionally qualified teacher of swimming, possessing a working knowledge of anatomy and physiology. If it is possible for both a physiotherapist and a swimming teacher to attend together this would be an ideal situation, for they could work in partnership and be of valuable help to each other. The person best suited to take charge would of course be one who is qualified both as a physiotherapist and a teacher of swimming.

Operation

1. The director briefs his assistants in the manner in which he intends to proceed.

2. The assistants enter the water and are delegated one to each pupil.

3. The director, working from the side of the pool, will instruct each assistant how to help his charge in a particular way, according to the prevailing disability.

4. As the lesson progresses, the director will move from one to another to confirm that his instructions are being followed and to note any characteristics that become apparent.

5. If both a teacher and physiotherapist are in attendance, the teacher, taking charge, will enable the physiotherapist to check limb track, resolution of force, body mechanics, etc. and to offer suggestions to the teacher in any situation that may arise.

6. The first few lessons should be of approximately fifteen minutes' duration. Paralytics feel the cold sooner than others, especially in the affected parts, and must be taken out of the water immediately they show any signs of discomfort and be made as warm and as comfortable as possible. As they become stronger, and their circulation improves, their period of time in the water will lengthen accordingly.

7. Introduce as a 'break' or, at the end of the lesson, a period of free play. The pupils enjoy this, and it enables them to become acquainted and have fun together as a relief from the monotony of exercise.

8. At the end of the session, director and assistants get together to discuss proceedings, to resolve any problems and to make constructive proposals and suggestions.

Here are some helpful suggestions for group teaching:

It is advisable for each assistant to remain with the same pupil for approximately six sessions and then to move to another pupil. In this way everybody becomes acquainted, and the assistants will gain experience and confidence with the various types of disability.

Award the pupils with a costume badge and certificate for endeavour and accomplishment, for swimming 20 yards or the length of the pool, for instance, or for any special endeavour enhanced by the degree of affliction. This, as well as being a compliment and reward, will boost morale immensely. The instinctive competitive element emerges and the pupils vie amongst themselves to emulate and surpass each other in greater effort. In addition to this, the fact of gaining their badge also places them on a footing with their more fortunate friends.

The physiotherapist can chart progress by physical development and performance out of the water, i.e. walking, arm swinging, etc., and the teacher by the quality of the stroke and the new skills acquired.

With the co-operation of the baths manager, the pool should be at the private disposal of the group. The average pool temperature should be constant at approximately 76° F. (25° C.), while the ideal for paralytics is approximately 90° F. (32° C.). The latter heat cannot, however, obtain where the pool is designed and intended for public use. Paralytics *must not* be taught in the open air, except in extremely warm and sunny climates.

Class teaching for the blind

I have used the heading 'class' in preference to 'group' in order to illustrate the difference between the two. In group teaching, there are several different abnormalities to be considered, and these, though taken collectively, are treated individually. In class teaching, on the other hand, each member is engaged in the same routine. The blind, though unfortunately unsighted, are not handicapped in the physical sense, so the appropriate director for such a class would be the teacher of swimming operating on the lines indicated for group teaching.

The assistants, eventually changing round to become familiar with each pupil, carry out the instructions of the director as in normal class instruction with each exercise being performed simultaneously. It would thus be possible to extend the size of the class to fifteen or twenty pupils. Being full of concentration, the blind are good and interested pupils, and there is no reason, as far as I am aware, why such a class should not attain success.

Note. Assistants must be very watchful, particularly in the early stages, that their pupils do not become submerged or swallow water through any oversight or neglect, and they should at all times, both in group and class teaching, speak quietly and instil all the confidence they possibly can.

Chapter VIII

SOME CASE HISTORIES

1. Jack W——, middle-aged. Dislocated (dorsal) vertebra in works accident.

After discharge from hospital he was unable to stoop properly or carry a light weight, e.g. attaché case. After learning to swim, his progress was rapid. Within a few months his spine became normal, and he can now, without any effort, carry his suitcases, do the gardening and is able to continue his occupation.

2. Ronnie G——, aged 14. Blind.

Learned to swim very quickly, with a very good action in all strokes. Swimming gave him immense confidence so that he went horse-riding and dancing. He is now a qualified masseur.

3. David R——, aged 12. Deaf and inarticulate.

As well as learning to swim, he was also receiving speech therapy. He, too, learned quickly the variety of strokes and developed a good style. For some time he was extremely shy and retiring, but gained plenty of confidence through being able to swim, and from his progress in speaking through speech therapy. He has overcome his shyness, travels on the Continent, and is now a cabinet-maker by trade.

4. John N——, aged 10. Has only one leg.

He was for a while very timid, until he learned to do a

forward glide. After that he made good progress, eventually passing a preliminary life-saving examination and is credited with effecting a canal rescue.

5. Alan B——, aged 12. Scoliosis.

Swims the lateral arm back stroke, but is not so comfortable with the surface arm back stroke, though his breast stroke is perfect.

Lessons were interrupted by surgical operations, yet he made steady progress and is now able to ride a motor-cycle.

6. Peter C——, aged 10. Hemiplegia.

A very happy boy. His left leg was badly affected, and this is one of the cases that responded to the 'splint' treatment described in the section on weakness of one side of the body on page 27. He is now able to walk without any aid and his arm is practically normal.

7. Alan L——, aged 13. Talipes Varus. Both feet badly affected.

Attended with his school for normal class instruction, and learned to swim during that period. He developed into a powerful breast stroke and life-saving back stroke swimmer, passing his life-saving examination at Medallion level. He much prefers these two strokes to the crawl, which he can only do for a short distance. His recovery was excellent. Cycling also helped a great deal and he is now an expert on skis.

8. Ian H——, aged 11. Hemiplegia, left side, leg very weak and wasted.

He swims the breast and surface arm back strokes, and

though his arm is very much stronger, his hand is still weak, especially in the region of the thumb. His leg is practically normal and it has assumed a full contour and he can now use it normally. He passed a test while swimming clothed, plays football, and runs the full course of two and a half miles in the school cross-country event.

9. John B——, aged 10. Spastic paraplegia, both legs.

Lessons were frequently interrupted by his absence due to minor ailments, and for a long time it was difficult during instruction to obtain his concentration. Anything would distract his attention, and it would be some time before I was able to resume with the lesson. It was eighteen months before he became water-borne. Progress was slow, as sometimes happens with this type of condition, but by perseverance, for he improved as he grew older, he is now able to swim several lengths breast stroke and there is a great improvement in his legs, which are now very much stronger, while the limp which was manifest in the beginning is now very much less so.

10. Harold W——, aged 30, farmer. Paralysis of both legs and of the left arm which was severely affected and wasted.

He was a well-built man weighing 188 lb., 6 ft. 2 in. in height, and had never been inside a baths building before. Being a much smaller man than he, I shall always admire his courage, for even in his helpless condition he resigned himself to me completely and with confidence. He made a wonderful recovery, walks now without any aid at all, drives a car and shares in all the work that farming entails. He possesses great and sincere faith as well as courage which, together with a cheerful personality, was a considerable help towards his ultimate and excellent recovery.

11. Geoffrey W——, aged 9. Scoliosis, and paralysis of the left leg and neck, which was practically immobile, and spasm of the abdominal muscles.

In poor physical shape, he was for some time confined to a wheelchair. Within four months he was swimming 25 yards life-saving back stroke, and a few yards breast stroke.

I then taught him somersaults in an endeavour to mobilize the neck muscles. This proved to be very effective and his muscles became stronger and his neck practically normal. As his swimming distance increased his legs also became much stronger, so that he was able to walk wearing a caliper. The scoliosis was being corrected and his abdominal muscles were more firm. His mother wrote: 'The specialist was very pleased with his general progress, with all-round improvement to the muscles, his scoliosis is being corrected, his neck muscles are much stronger, and he has had a new support ring to his caliper owing to the amazing development to the paralysed leg.'

As his physical condition improved, so did his confidence and academic ability, so that ultimately he passed his entrance examination to a grammar school, and later to a university.

The following press announcement records a happy sequel.

'Polio victim is still winning battles'

'A former —— grammar school pupil, Geoffrey W——, a polio victim, who has won his battle to walk without the aid of crutches, has passed his second-year examination for his Bachelor of Law degree at —— University. He was stricken down with polio when eight years old, but passed his grammar school entrance examination after being given special instruction from his mother.'

A great triumph for himself and his devoted parents who did so much to help with his studies, when as a young boy his absence from school was enforced. Throughout my association with him, he displayed wonderful fortitude and patience. His reward is well deserved.

Chapter IX

A TYPICAL SEQUENCE OF LESSONS AND EXERCISES

These were adopted for the teaching of Harold W——, referred to in Case History 10 on page 65.

My first impression of Harold was of a man in normal health, of powerful physique, with a well-proportioned and cared-for body.

The attack of poliomyelitis had affected both legs and his left arm which were rendered useless, his only sound limb being his right arm, which was well developed and strong.

Regarding his legs and toes, which he was unable to move, I did not notice much wasting of flesh in any particular region, but his left arm was greatly affected. There were signs of much wasting, especially in the region of the deltoid, trapezius and pectoral groups. The arm was very thin, with little evidence of the presence of the triceps and biceps, whilst the muscles of the thumb were wasted and useless. These were my observations, and my analysis was that the patient, never having been in the water before and having no power to balance, would have to be instructed in back stroke swimming, the main object being to inspire confidence, and to help him to acquire balance in the water, to mobilize and strengthen his legs, and to develop an arm stroke in order to exercise his arms. Placing my hands under his arm-pits I towed him along on his back, allowing him to get the feel of the water, and to get acclimatized to his new surroundings, at the same time keeping up a conversation to induce a feeling of relaxation and to gain his confidence.

He was naturally buoyant, and when I explained how to float with his hands clasped on his chest, he managed it without trouble, although there was a tendency to dip the left shoulder a little. He soon learned how to balance in this position and also with his arms by his sides. This natural ability was an immensely useful factor in the exercises that were to follow. Supporting him under the arm-pits, I got him to drop his hips, submerging the legs, and then to move them up and down in a back crawl fashion (*see* Fig. 15). The ability to do this increased his confidence, and with it, a sense of hope.

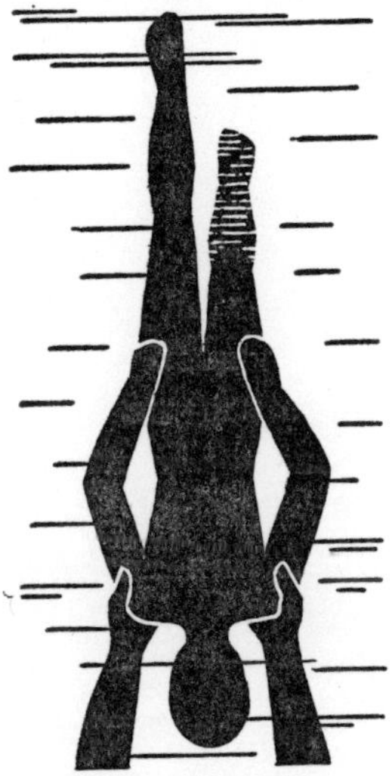

15. A pupil who had had poliomyelitis, supported under the arm-pits and performing the back crawl leg kick

Before leaving the pool I towed him to where the water was 5 ft. deep, and he was able to stand up. Holding both his hands I walked backwards in front of him, and he took three or four steps forward. I did not persist in this on his first two or three visits, but cultivated it by degrees. Having gained confidence and relaxation in my pupil, I began to teach him the life-saving back stroke kick, with the arms folded or resting on the chest, and supported him until he acquired the movement.

I now resorted to the 'pull-rope', which has a linen sling approximately 4 in. wide attached to one end, and a rubber ring support (*see* Fig. 16). Placing the sling around his chest,

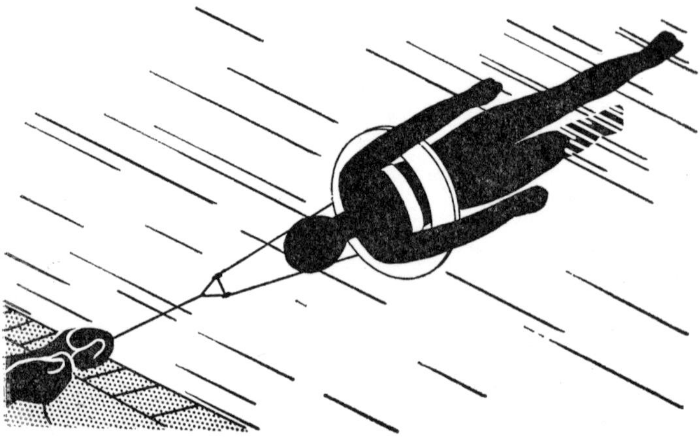

16. The same patient as in Fig. 15 learns the back stroke with the aid of a 'pull-rope' and rubber ring support

and the ring support under his arm-pits, I stood on the side of the pool and, by pulling on the rope, assisted him to swim the back stroke, at the same time emphasizing the movements of the legs, particularly the push with the soles of the feet and the extension of the legs. As the stroke improved I lessened the pull on the rope until eventually I had no need to exert a pull at all. At this stage I removed the sling and the ring support to replace it with a 'loop' support.

I have found this loop support to be very useful. It is a converted bicycle inner tube simply tied in the middle to form two loops. When swimming on the front, the pupil wears it across the back with the loops resting on the shoulders, and reversed when swimming on the back (*see* Fig. 17). Unlike the conventional ring support, it does not encumber or restrict the arms, the body does not ride so high in the water and approximates more to a swimming posture. Using the loop support only, and without any assistance from me,

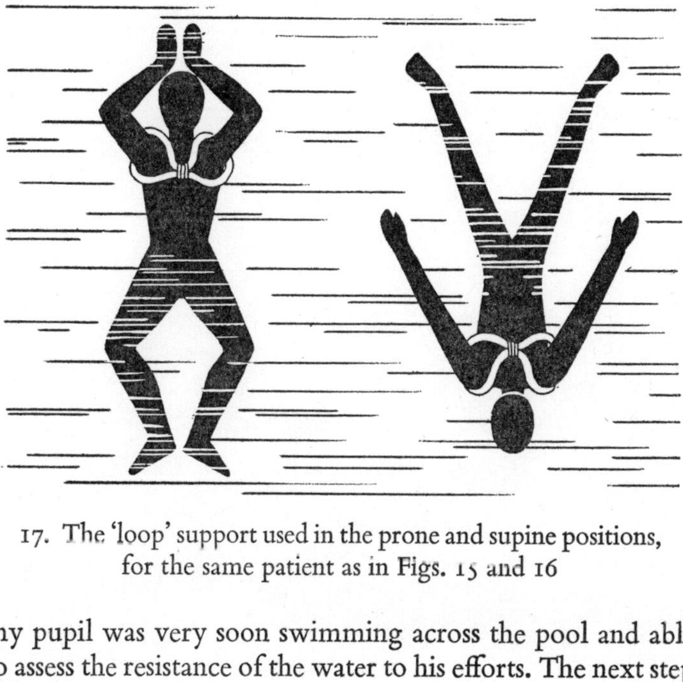

17. The 'loop' support used in the prone and supine positions, for the same patient as in Figs. 15 and 16

my pupil was very soon swimming across the pool and able to assess the resistance of the water to his efforts. The next step was to remove the support entirely and, with the aid of the pull-rope, I again assisted him until he was able to manage without a pull from me. Soon, after swimming across the pool on his own, he was able to swim the length of the pool, and subsequently the distance was increased with practice. Lessons were interspersed with exercises, i.e. knee flexors and extensors and hip flexors and extensors, as well as encouragement to walk shoulder high in the water, holding hands and later held by the tips of the fingers, till at last he could walk without my assistance.

After walking about 6 yards his right leg would give way and he had to halt. By degrees his legs got stronger and he was able to walk across the pool at this depth without fault. When he could do this with ease and comfort, I took him into shallower water, chest high, until he could accomplish the same exercise.

It must be appreciated that these processes were only gradual and coincided with his regular visits, and during this time I concentrated on his utilizing the back stroke only in an effort to recover the use of his legs. The next effort was to try to walk from the deep to the shallow end of the pool, which would give proof of the strength of his legs. He did very well until he was waist-deep, when again his leg would collapse and a halt was made. His left leg was strengthening more quickly than his right, and during swimming exercises we paid a lot of attention to the right leg, as well as to feet exercises in deep water, i.e. raising and lowering the heels, hopping off one foot and then the other to strengthen the toes and extensors. Eventually he walked unaided the length of the pool from the deep to the shallow end, but it was some time before he could walk to and fro across the shallow end without experiencing difficulty. Within three months of his first visit he was swimming 75 yards, while the walking exercises in the water were progressing well. Instead of arriving on a stretcher in the usual way, wearing calipers and supporting himself with his arms round the shoulders of the ambulance attendants, he now walked into the building to be independent of the stretcher for ever.

I now introduced the lateral arm movement to the back

stroke, my main theme being to mobilize the shoulders and arms in an endeavour later to extend the radius of the arm movement. The rudiments of this stroke were soon mastered, the distance increased and the legs became more powerful. During the arm stroke it was observed that the left arm had little power and the water could be seen pushing the fingers back. I would walk alongside him and increase the resistance by making him press against my fingers as the hand was brought to the side (*see* Fig. 18).

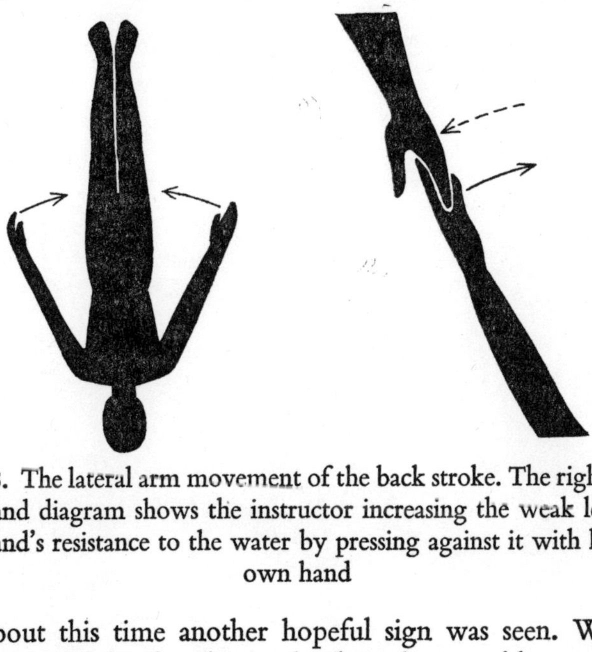

18. The lateral arm movement of the back stroke. The right-hand diagram shows the instructor increasing the weak left hand's resistance to the water by pressing against it with his own hand

About this time another hopeful sign was seen. Whilst dressing with his feet flat on the floor, he was able to move, though only very slightly, the extensor of his left foot and his toes showed signs of movement for the first time, though the right foot still remained inactive. I now sought to extend the radius of the arm movement by introducing the surface arm back stroke, and demonstrated the stroke to give a picture of what I wanted.

I guided his left arm in the exercise while he responded with his right, but a problem arose when he came to swim the stroke alone, for beyond bending his left arm with the hand close to the neck, he was unable to extend it further. This was overcome by his gripping the fingers of the left hand with his right hand and extending the arms to the required position beyond the head (*see* Fig. 19), holding the position for an appreciable time and gently stretching the arms during this period. The pull downwards had already been acquired from the earlier stroke which formed part of the main theme.

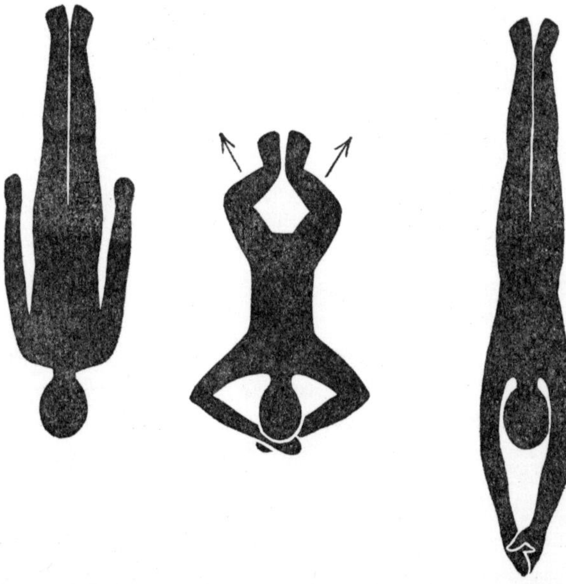

19. The surface arm back stroke. The pupil extends his weak left arm beyond his head by gripping the fingers of the left hand with the right hand

Gradually and with practice the left arm could be extended to a position 2 or 3 in. beyond the head. From this point we introduced a 'flick' to try and make the left arm less dependent on the right. As the left arm reached its position 2 or 3 in. beyond the head, the flick was made by the fingers of the right hand smartly striking the backs of the fingers of the left, causing the hand and arm to slide into the extended position beyond the head. This gave the feeling of pushing with the left hand and arm, and as the push improved and increased the flick was gradually reduced, until the movement was mastered without any assistance, and he was able to travel two or three lengths of the pool without any signs of discomfort.

We now added to the exercises for the legs and feet exercises for the shoulders, arms and fingers, alternating these with the others. Very good progress was maintained, as can be gauged by the following observations. The caliper from the right leg was discarded, the left one retained, and with the patient using a walking-stick in the right hand, an attendant was no longer needed. Formerly, when sitting down at a table, he had been unable to place his left hand upon it without assistance from the right hand. He could now place his elbow on the table with ease. The breast stroke was now introduced and, due to the back stroke training, no problem was encountered with the legs, so to initiate the arm stroke I once more resorted to the pull-rope and ring support (*see* Fig. 20).

In this stroke the left arm would not move forward under its own power due to the reverse position of the body and to the lack of strength in the arm to press on the water in order to maintain the balance of the body. We therefore adopted a similar method of extending the arm as in the surface arm back stroke. Whilst in the 'crouch' position, the fingers of the left hand were placed on top of the fingers of the right hand and carried forward to the extended position.

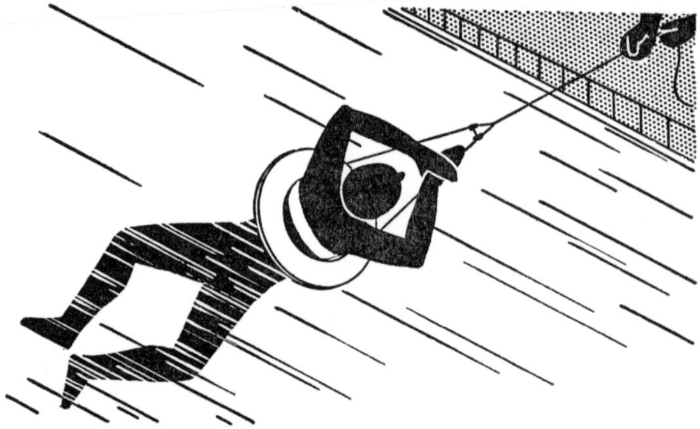

20. The breast stroke. The weak left hand is placed on the right and carried forward to the extended position

When using the loop support, he could keep his arm straight during the 'press' position and recover his arm easily, but on removing the support and using the pull-rope only, his balance immediately became affected after the 'crouch' position, due to the lack of power in the left hand and arm. He could not get the required 'press' to maintain his balance, so for the time being we used a 'trick' press, that is, with the arm held in a bent position, using the elbow for power. Even then, the position could only be held for a brief period before the arm had to recover, and during the recovery movement the hand and forearm would 'feather' in a lateral movement to the chest, and for a time there was a dipping of the left shoulder. This was eliminated to a great extent by depressing the right shoulder, and this later helped in improving the action of the left arm. To assist the left arm we also used a small wooden block measuring approximately 4 in. by 3 in. by ½ in. and the block was held flat and lengthwise in the left hand and the increased resistance cultivated a stronger 'press'.

He now manages on his own to swim 25 yards breast stroke, but the above characteristics are still present, and the left hand still has to be guided to its forward position, but rather more from a frontal angle than from the chest as in the beginning and as the stroke is influenced by the left arm to a great degree, it is necessary to swim with the head up which brings a crick to the neck.

Breathing out with the face submerged has been tried without success, so until the arm becomes stronger we must persevere and for a time be content. Strokes are alternated during swims up and down the pool, beginning with the lateral arm back stroke, and changing to the surface arm back stroke, breast stroke, and back stroke without the use of the arms. The limbs are getting stronger, movement is returning, the toes which were originally unable to move can now twiddle, and his fingers are beginning to move to a slight degree. Apart from his swimming, which continues to improve, he can travel by the 'propellor' a distance of 20 yards, surface dive and recover an object in 5½ ft. of water. This, then, is the degree of progress at the end of twelve months, and we are hopeful that by continuing this programme we shall achieve ultimate success and be able to look forward to perhaps even greater recovery.

Chapter X

THE FUTURE

With the building of more swimming pools by local councils and school authorities, the teaching of swimming to the physically handicapped will become more widespread, and with this in mind I propose the following recommendations with regard to the important features of pool construction.

THE LEARNERS' POOL

This should be used solely for private tuition. It must be contained within its own four walls and completely separated from the open public pool. The advantages of this are both psychological and physical (*see* Fig. 21).

Dimensions

The pool should measure approximately 45 ft. by 24 ft., shelving from 3 ft. to 5 ft. deep.

Construction

The floor of the pool should be covered with suitable non-slip tiles.

The exercise rail

If an overflow channel surrounds the pool, an exercise rail

should be fixed to the wall at the shallow end at water level, so that a pupil can either under-grasp the rail with the hands, or tuck the feet under the rail, positions that are necessary for the performance of certain exercises.

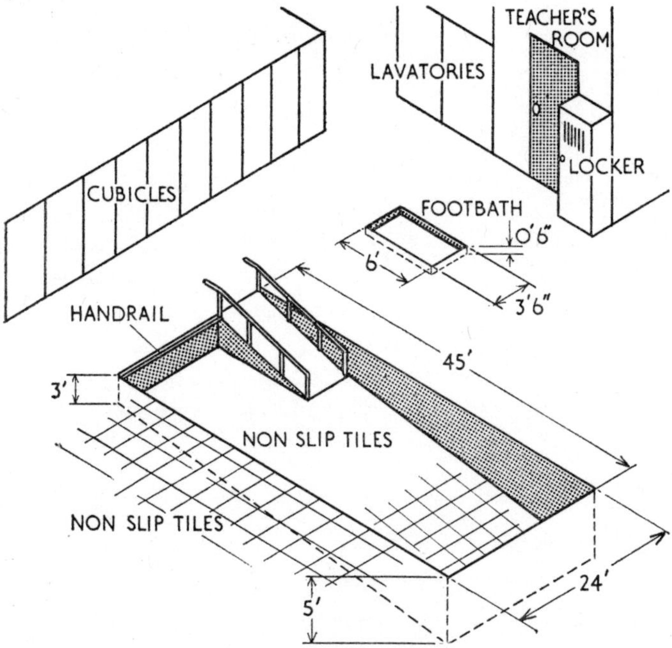

21. Diagram of the learners' pool

The pool surround

The floor should again be covered with suitable non-slip tiles, and should be wide enough to give free passage to a wheelchair.

The ramp

For safe and easy access to and from the water, this should

be covered with a non-slip material, and fitted with a double hand-rail.

Cubicles and toilets

These should for convenience be sited on the pool surround.

The foot bath

An asset is an outsize footbath, approximately 6 ft. by $3\frac{1}{2}$ ft. by 6 in. deep. As well as fulfilling its intended purpose, it can also be used as a place of rest by those who soon get tired and over-exerted, where they can relax and recuperate in warmth and comfort. It is also most useful for exercising the limbs of very young children, from 3 to 4 years old. The child's head is rested on a rubber float, and the teacher can quite conveniently guide the limbs through various exercises.

The teacher's accommodation

The teacher should have a private dressing-room where his clothes will be in a comparatively dry atmosphere, instead of in a cubicle open to the humid atmosphere of the pool. His dressing-room should be sited on the pool surround, and fitted with a desk and cupboards, etc., so that all necessary clerical work can be done on the spot.

A cupboard or locker

This item should be sited on the pool surround, where the teacher can store his equipment such as swimming aids and other accessories. These articles of equipment are most important, since they are the tools of his trade and usually they have to be transported to another part of the building where they are open to access, within the reach of all, and they are very often mislaid. A place in which to store them is therefore essential.

In a pool designed as I have described, the swimming teacher has the means of being of the greatest service to physically handicapped children, who often feel that they have not had a 'square deal' from life. When they learn to swim, they achieve something of immeasurable value, and their efforts are amply rewarded. No longer are they despondent, frustrated and alone; they are now 'in the swim'. Almost immediately their outlook brightens, their interests broaden, their academic work improves, and they become increasingly independent and self-reliant. Independence begets confidence. This confidence grows with maturity and enables them to earn their living, to sustain themselves and, from what appeared at first to be a hopeless and forlorn beginning, to pursue an active and effective life.

Not one of all the pupils I have taught could originally swim. All of them were required to attend for periodical medical checks, but as a result of their instruction it was not found necessary for any of them to attend for clinical exercises. All were told, 'Keep on with your swimming,' and this is the finest testimonial to the type of instruction I have described.

INDEX

INDEX